Paleo Cookbook for Two

Everyday Delicious and Healthy Recipes!

Disclaimer and Terms of Use:

Effort has been made to ensure that the information in this book is accurate and complete, however, the author and the publisher do not warrant the accuracy of the information, text and graphics contained within the book due to the rapidly changing nature of science, research, known and unknown facts and internet. The Author and the publisher do not hold any responsibility for errors, omissions or contrary interpretation of the subject matter herein. This book is presented solely for motivational and informational purposes only.

What This Book is All About

Are you having difficulty about what Paleo meal to cook every day for yourself and your loved one? Do you have fear that you might both wander away from a healthy diet routine you have started merely because you lack options? Making a healthy meal for two every day can become a complicated task. However, you don't have to worry anymore! This book is perfect for you as it provides 50 scrumptious Paleo recipes that will be perfect just for two. If you will be having a couple guests over, you can just double the ingredients and you'll have mouthwatering, healthy food served on your table.

Did you know that a Paleo diet is one of the most effective ways of consuming a healthy food? The nutritious and unrefined food in this diet ensures you stay healthy, strong, toxic-free and active. The most significant benefit of this diet is that it helps prevent diseases, such as diabetes, obesity, and many others, because it contains healthy options.

This book contains 50 Paleo recipes for two, which are easy to make, including:

a) List of Paleo food items
b) Recipes for different categories of meals i.e. Breakfast, Main Course, Dessert etc.
c) Step by step easy instructions

Start making these delicious and healthy meals today!

Contents

Introduction

The Paleo Diet is also known as "Primal" "Whole Food" or "Ancestral" diet. It is a modernized diet plan that stems from the Paleolithic Era's ancient diet, which is a period that lasted 2.5 million years and came to its end about 10,000 years ago with the initiation of agriculture. This diet is based on modern everyday food items, which mimic those food items eaten in prehistoric times. According to this diet, people must consume unprocessed, grain-free and real food in order to stay fit.

Supporters of Paleo diet state that quality of food preparation and cultivation declined greatly about 10,000 years ago. This was due to the advent of domestication of animals and agriculture. The supports also argue that human beings have not properly evolved to digest newer foods like dairy, legumes and grain much less the calorie loaded and high processed foods which is now cheaply and readily available in the market. This food is the cause of leading health problems like diabetes, heart disease and obesity. Many researches in dermatology, ophthalmology, biochemistry, biology and other disciplines indicate that the modern diet, which consists of sugar, trans fats and refined food, also is the cause for infertility, depression, Alzheimer's, Parkinson's and cancer.

According to the health critics, the Paleo Diet can help individuals to lead a healthier, longer and active life. This diet has gained a buzzing popularity among the health conscious people all over the world. This is considered to be the healthiest approach to eating healthy because the nutrition from this diet is still hardwired into our genetics. Paleo diet is the most healthy and nutritional approach, which perfectly works with human genetics and helps in staying energetic, strong and lean.

This diet will help you stay slender, tough, and full of energy. However, as many diet plans have restrictions, a Paleo Diet does as well, there are certain things that you can eat and some that you can't. Here is a short version list of what to eat and what not to eat on a Paleo diet:

Things you can Eat in Paleo Diet

Things to eat include:

1. Fresh Vegetables,
2. Seeds,
3. Fish/seafood,
4. Eggs,
5. Fresh fruits,
6. Grass-produced meats,
7. Nuts,
8. Oils (coconut, avocado, macadamia, flaxseed, walnut, and olive).

Things You can't Eat in Paleo Diet

Things not to eat include:

1. Refined sugar,

2. Potatoes,
3. Candy / Junk / Processed Food,
4. Cereal grains,
5. Salt,
6. Processed foods,
7. Dairy,
8. Legumes (including peanuts),
9. Refined vegetable oils.

Paleo Food List

Meats

Lamb Rack, Chicken Wings, Chicken Leg, Chicken Thigh, Chicken Breast, Turkey, Grass Fed Beef, Ground Beef, Pork, Pork Tenderloin, Pork Chops, Steak, Bacon, Poultry, Bison, Shrimp, Veal, New York Steak, Buffalo, Lobster, Venison, Steaks, Salmon, Clams, Rattlesnake, Chuck Steak, Quail, Lean Veal, Pheasant, Ostrich, Bison Steaks, Turtle, Reindeer, Wild Boar, Eggs (duck, chicken or goose), Bison Jerky, Beef Jerky, Bison Rib eye, Bison Sirloin, Bear, Lamb Chops, Kangaroo, Rabbit, Goose, Emu, Elk, Goat.

Sea Food

Lobster, Halibut, Scallops, Clams, Shrimp, Oysters, Crayfish, Salmon, Mackerel, Trout, Bass, Walleye, Crawfish, Swordfish, Sardines, Tuna, Red Snapper, Shark, Sunfish, Crab, Tilapia.

Fruits

Plums, Pineapple, Watermelon, Persimmon, Tangerine, Pears, Strawberries, Peaches, Star Fruit, Passion Fruit, Rhubarb, Papaya, Raspberries, Orange, Pomegranate, Nectarine, Mango, Cherries, Lychee, Cherimoya, Lime, Melon, Cassava, Lemon, Carambola, Kiwi, Cantaloupe, Honeydew melon, Boysenberries, Guava Blueberries, Blackberries, Grapes, Grapefruit, Banana, Gooseberries, Avocado, Apricot, Cranberries, Apple, Figs.

Vegetables

Artichoke, Mushrooms, Asparagus, Mustard Greens, Beet Greens, Onions, Beets, Parsley, Bell Peppers, Parsnip, Broccoli, Peppers (all kinds), Brussels Sprouts, Pumpkin, Cabbage, Purslane, Carrots, Radish, Cauliflower, Rutabaga, Celery, Seaweed, Collards, Spinach, Cucumber, Squash (all kinds), Dandelion, Swiss Chard, Eggplant, Tomatillos, Endive, Tomato, Green Onions, Turnip Greens, Kale, Turnips, Kohlrabi, Watercress, Lettuce.

Nuts and Seeds

Almonds, Pine Nuts, Brazil Nuts, Pistachios (unsalted), Cashews, Pumpkin Seeds, Chestnuts, Sesame Seeds, Hazelnuts, Sunflower Seeds, Macadamia Nuts, Walnuts, Pecans.

Oils

Coconut Oil, Olive Oil, Macadamia Oil, Avocado Oil, Grass fed Butter.

Paleo Pancakes

Ingredients

Almond flour – 1 cup

Fresh berries – 1 cup

Coconut oil – 1 tsp

Sea Salt – ¼ tsp

Nutmeg – ¼ tsp (grated)

Water – ¼ cup

Unsweetened applesauce – ½ cup

Eggs – 2

Coconut flour – 1 tbsp

Instructions

1. In a bowl, mix together sea salt, nutmeg, eggs, coconut flour, applesauce and almond flour. Mix till it appears thicker as compared to a normal mix.
2. Pour coconut oil in a saucepan and put on medium heat. Once it is heated, Spoon ¼ cup batter on the pan and spread out if needed.
3. When bubbles start appearing on the top, flip to the other side and let it cook for 1-2 minutes.
4. Take out and place it on a plate.
5. Repeat this process and make a stack on pancakes on two plates.
6. Once the batter is finished and all the pancakes have been made, top them up with fresh berries and serve.

Sausage Omelet with Roasted Peppers

Ingredients

Bell pepper – 2

Eggs – 4

Ground black pepper – 1 tsp

Coconut oil – 2 tsp

Pork Sausage – ½ lb (cooked and sliced)

Parsley – 2 tbsp (chopped)

Instructions

1. Place a heavy bottomed pan on stove on high heat. Place the peppers in. When the skin of the peppers starts blackening on either side, remove them from pan.
2. Place the peppers in a plastic bag with a sprinkle of water. Seal the bag and put it aside for 5 minutes. Afterwards, take out the peppers remove their skin and seeds, and then dice them.
3. In a bowl, beat eggs mixed with black pepper.
4. Add coconut oil in a skillet on medium heat.
5. Pour in half egg mixture in the skillet and when they start to set, add half of the sliced sausages, peppers and parsley on one side of the omelet.
6. When the mixture is fully set, fold the half of the omelet over the filling.
7. Repeat the process with the other half of the egg mixture for the second omelet.

Eggs with Paleo Steak

Ingredients

Boneless beefsteak – ½ lb (sliced)

Eggs – 2

Spinach – 1 handful

Red bell pepper – 1 (diced)

Yellow onion – ¼ (diced)

Mushrooms – 4 (sliced)

Coconut oil – 2 tsp

Sea salt – ¼ tsp

Black pepper – ¼ tsp

Instructions

1. Season the beef with black pepper and salt.
2. On medium-high heat, place a sauté pan and add coconut oil, beef, mushrooms and onions.
3. Sauté them till the beefsteak is a little cooked.
4. Add in spinach and bell pepper. Cook till the beef is done.
5. In a frying pan, add some coconut oil and fry the eggs.
6. Take out two plates. Divide the veggies and beef steak on them and top with fried eggs.
7. Serve hot.

Cinnamon Fruit Salad

Ingredients

Orange – 1 (peeled and diced)

Apple – 1 (diced)

Walnuts or pecans – ½ cup (chopped)

Cinnamon – ½ tsp

Instructions

1. In a bowl, add all the fruits.
2. Top with cinnamon and nuts.
3. Serve.

Delicious Paleo Muffins

Ingredients

Almond flour – 1 cup

Coconut flour – ½ cup

Tapioca flour – ½ cup

Baking soda – 2 tsp

Sea salt – 1 tsp

Allspice – 1 tbsp

Cinnamon – 1 tbsp

Dates – 1 cup (pitted)

Ripe bananas – 3

Eggs – 3

Apple cider vinegar – 1 tsp

Coconut oil – ¼ cup

Fresh berries – 1 ¼ cup

Zucchini – ¾ cup (grated)

Almonds – ¾ (chopped)

Instructions

1. Put your oven on preheat on 350°F
2. Mix together, all spice, cinnamon, salt, baking soda, tapioca flour, coconut flour and almond flour in a bowl.
3. Combine oil, vinegar, eggs, bananas and dates in a food processor.
4. Pour all these mixtures in a big bowl. Mix till combined.
5. Take zucchini and grate it finely.
6. Mix together almonds, zucchini and berries.
7. Spoon this mixture into muffin trays and bake for 20 minutes.
8. Serve warm.

Eggs with Veggies

Ingredients

Bacon – 4 strips

Yellow onion – ¼ (diced)

Spinach leaves – handful (chopped)

Garlic – 1 clove (minced)

Eggs – 4

Avocado – 1 (sliced)

Instructions

1. In a pan, heat oil and start cooking bacon. Once it is done, remove the bacon from the pan. Using a paper towel, absorb any extra oil from the bacon.
2. Crumble the bacon, set aside to let it cool.
3. Save 4 tbsp of bacon grease and drain the rest of the pan.
4. In the bacon grease, sauté the onions till translucent. Include garlic and cook till tender.
5. Separate this mixture in two plates.
6. Cook eggs in the grease left on the pan. Once cooked, add them on top of the veggies on each plate.
7. Place sliced avocado over them and top with crumbled bacon.

Paleo Bacon Rings

Ingredients

Bacon – 6 strips

Eggs – 4

Tomato – 1 (sliced in 4 pieces)

Onion – 1/3 cup (chopped)

Mushrooms – 4 (chopped)

Ground black pepper – ½ tsp

Instructions

1. Put your oven on preheat at 325°F
2. Put a skillet on medium heat and cook bacon for 3 minutes or until it starts shriveling. Set it aside.
3. Save a small amount of bacon fat from the skillet and discard the rest.
4. Brush the bacon fat on 2 muffin cups or small ramekins.
5. With the left over bacon drippings, cook mushrooms and onions on a pan over medium heat till they soften.
6. In the cups or ramekins, add a tomato slice at the bottom.
7. Include bacon strips in both cups.
8. Top the muffin cup with an egg and sprinkle pepper.
9. Add onions and mushrooms on the egg.
10. Place the ramekins or muffin tray in the oven for 20 minutes. (Note: Cover the empty cups on the muffin tray with water to prevent burning)
11. Once they are done, with a spatula carefully loosen the egg edges and transfer them in to plates.
12. Serve hot.

Bacon, Eggies and Veggies

Ingredients

Bacon – 4 slices

Eggs – 4

Zucchini – 1 (diced)

Garlic – 1 clove (minced)

Tomato – 1 (diced)

Spinach leaves- handful

Instructions

1. In a pan, cook bacon. Once done, set it aside. Keep 1 tbsp of bacon grease and drain the rest.
2. In the bacon grease, add tomato, garlic and zucchini and sauté till about to become tender.
3. In a clean bowl, beat eggs.
4. Crumble the bacon.
5. When the veggies are done, add crumbled bacon and beaten eggs in the pan. Sprinkle spinach leaves on top.
6. Cook on medium low heat till eggs are firm and fluffy.
7. Serve warm.

Stir-fry Sausages

Ingredients

Coconut oil – 1 tsp

Yellow onion – ½ (diced)

Sausages – ½ lb (sliced)

Spinach– 4 cups

Instructions

1. Heat coconut oil in a skillet on medium heat.
2. Sauté onions till translucent. Include sausages. Toss them frequently and cook till brown.
3. Add spinach. Lower the heat and cover.
4. After about 5 minutes or till the greens are soft. Remove from heat.
5. Serve warm.

Stir-fry Chicken

Ingredients

Eggs – 2

Water – 1 tbsp

Coconut oil – 1 tsp

Asparagus – ¼ lb (washed and cut in 2" pieces)

Red bell pepper – 1 (sliced)

Garlic – 1 clove (minced)

Chicken breast – ½ lb (cooked and diced)

Olives – ½ cup (sliced)

Almonds – ¼ cup

Avocado – ½ (sliced)

Sea salt – to taste

Instructions

1. Beat eggs in a bowl and mix water.
2. Add oil in a skillet on medium high speed. Add garlic, red pepper and asparagus. Sauté till they become tender.
3. Include olives, eggs and chicken. Cook till tender, stirring continuously. Ensure the chicken has been heated through and the eggs are cooked.
4. Sprinkle sea salt and top with avocado and almonds.

Mushroom Creamy Soup

Ingredients

Avocados – 2 (pitted and peeled)

Grapefruit juice – 1 cup

Garlic – 1 clove

Hot water – 2 cups

Coconut oil – 1 tbsp

Mushrooms – 1 cup (sliced)

Red sweet pepper – 1 (diced)

Yellow onion – ¼ (minced)

Tomatoes – 2 (diced)

Basil – 4 sprigs

Instructions

1. Blend together water, garlic, grapefruit juice and avocado in a food processor and set aside.
2. In a pan, heat coconut oil. Sauté basil, tomato, onion, sweet pepper and mushrooms till they soften.
3. Pour in the avocado mixture.
4. Transfer the soup in a bowl.
5. Serve hot.

Veggies Soup

Ingredients

Coconut oil – 2 tbsp

Yellow onion – ½ (diced)

Carrots – 2 (sliced)

Zucchini – 2 (sliced)

Parsley – 4 sprigs (chopped)

Thyme – ½ tsp dried or 2 sprigs fresh

Ground pepper and sea salt – to taste

Vegetable broth – 4 cups

Instructions

1. In a pan, heat coconut oil and cook onion till translucent.
2. Include carrots, zucchini, parsley, thyme, pepper and salt. Cover the pan.
3. Cook for 10 minutes on low heat till veggies are tender.
4. Pour in the vegetable stock and turn the heat up. When the mixture boils, lower the heat to medium.
5. Cook for 20 minutes or till veggies become soft.
6. Serve hot.

Chicken Curry Coconut Soup

Ingredients

Coconut oil – 1 tbsp

Onion – 1 (chopped)

Garlic – 1 clove (minced)

Cauliflower – 1 cup (chopped)

Curry powder – 1 tbsp

Ground cumin – 1 tsp

Chicken broth – 4 cups

Chicken – 3 cups (cooked and shredded)

Lime juice – 2 tbsp

Coconut milk – 1 can

Cilantro – for garnish (chopped)

Salt and ground pepper – to taste

Instructions

1. Heat a soup pot and add coconut oil.
2. Cook onion till they soften.
3. Add cauliflower and garlic. Cook for 5 minutes and include all the spices.
4. After stirring for 1 minute, add the chicken stock.
5. Let it cook for 10 minutes on low heat.
6. Add coconut milk, lime juice and chicken.
7. Let it cook for a few minute and pour in a bowl.
8. Top it with cilantro and coconut flakes. Serve.

Classic Paleo Bone Broth

Ingredients

Chicken necks, wings and bones – 2 lbs

Yellow onion – 1 (chopped)

Mixed vegetables – 4 cups (chopped)

Bay leaves – 2

Black peppercorns – 1 tbsp

Oregano – 1 tbsp

Fennel seed – 1 tbsp

Thyme – 1 tsp

Sea salt – 2 tbsp

Apple cider vinegar – 2 tbsp

Water – as needed

Instructions

1. Put oven on preheat at 350 °F.
2. Roast the bones for 20 minutes.
3. Once done transfer the bones in a large soup pot. Add all the ingredients. Pour in water and fill the pot.
4. Cover and cook for 7-24 hours.
5. Serve hot.

Summertime Cold Soup

Ingredients

Tomato – 4 (quartered)

Onion – 1 (chopped)

Cucumber – 1 (chopped)

Parsley – 1 sprig

Garlic – 1 clove (peeled)

Cold water – ½ cup

Lemon juice – 1 lemon

Sea salt – to taste

Black pepper – to taste

Cayenne – 1 (chopped)

Ice cubes – 4

Instructions

1. Mix these ingredients together in a food processor.
2. Serve cold.

Paleo Salads

Sauté Cashew and Chard

Ingredients

Swiss chard – 1 bunch (strips)

Cashews – ½ cup

Olive oil – 1 tbsp

Sea salt – to taste

Ground black pepper – to taste

Instructions

1. On medium heat, place a skillet and pour olive oil.
2. Add cashews and chard in the skittle. Sauté till leaves start to wilt.
3. Season with salt and pepper.
4. Serve hot.

Tunalicious Salad

Ingredients

Tuna – 2 cans

Black olives – 1 cup (chopped)

Green onions – 2 (chopped)

Jalapeno pepper – 1 (finely chopped)

Red chili flakes – ½ tsp

Lemon juice – 2 lemons

Olive oil – 2 tsp

Lettuce – 1 head

Avocado – 1 (sliced)

Instructions

1. Combine tuna, olives, onions, jalapeno, lemon juice and olive oil. Mix well.
2. Serve over lettuce.
3. Top with avocado and sprinkle red chili flakes.

Waldorf Chicken Salad

Ingredients

Chicken breasts – 2 (cooked and diced)

Apple – 1 (diced)

Stalk celery – 1 (chopped)

Walnuts – ½ cup (chopped)

Mayonnaise – ¼ cup

Lime juice – 2 tsp

Raw honey – 2 tsp

Ground black pepper – to taste

Sea salt – to taste

Instructions

1. Mix together walnuts, celery, apple and chicken in a bowl and set aside.
2. In a smaller bowl, mix honey, lime juice and mayonnaise till blended together.
3. Sprinkle pepper and salt.
4. Pour the dressing on the chicken and give it a toss to mix well.

Taco Paleo Salad

Ingredients

Ground beef – 1 lb

Chili powder – 2 tbsp

Garlic salt – 1 tsp

Oregano – ½ tsp

Sea salt – ½ tsp

Water – ¾ cup

Yellow onion – ½ (diced)

Tomato – 1 (diced)

Romaine heart lettuce – 3

Black olives – 1 can (sliced)

Avocado – 1 (sliced)

Fresh cilantro – as required

Salsa – 1 jar

Instructions

1. On medium high heat, place a skillet and add beef in it. Include onion and cook till it turns brown.
2. Include water, salt, oregano, cumin, garlic salt and chili powder. Cook for 5 minutes.
3. Wash the lettuce carefully tear them and place on two plates.
4. Place the beef mixture on the lettuce. Top with salsa, tomatoes, avocado, cilantro and black olives.

Fajita Chicken Salad

Ingredients

Coconut oil – 1 tbsp

Yellow onion – ½ (diced)

Chicken breasts – ½ lb (skinless and boneless)

Cumin – ½ tsp

Dried oregano – 2 tsp

Sea salt – ¼ tsp

Bell pepper – 1 (chopped)

Romaine Lettuce – 1

Tomatoes – 2 (diced)

Avocado – 1 (sliced)

Instructions

1. Cut the skinless and boneless chicken in 2" slices.
2. Place a skillet on high heat; add coconut oil and sauté onions till translucent and soft.
3. Include salt, oregano, cumin and chicken. Cook till brown, stirring occasionally.
4. Include peppers and let it cook till they become tender.
5. Shred the lettuce and place in two plates.
6. Place the chicken mix over them.
7. Top with avocado and tomatoes.

Paleo Seafood

Plaice fillets and almond with crust

Ingredients

Plaice fillets – 1 lb

Almond flour – 1 cup

Sea salt – to taste

Ground black pepper – to taste

Egg – 1 (beaten)

Coconut oil – 1 tbsp

Instructions

1. In a bowl, mix together pepper, salt and almond flour.
2. Wash the fillets and pat dry.
3. Dip fillets in beaten egg mixture and then in almond flour mixture, making sure that the fillet is coated completely.
4. Heat a skillet on high heat and pour in the coconut oil.
5. Fry one fillet at a time, 3 minutes each side.
6. Place them on two plates and serve hot.

Halibut, Balsamic and Vegetables

Ingredients

<u>For Veggies:</u>

Sweet potato – 1 (cubed)

Red pepper – 1 (diced)

Yellow pepper – 1 (diced)

Olive oil – 1 tbsp

Balsamic vinegar – 1 tsp

Spinach leaves – 2 cups

<u>For Halibut:</u>

Halibut filets – 2 (6-8 ounce)

Cumin – 1 tsp

Olive oil – 1 tbsp

Instructions

1. Put your oven on preheat for 400 °F.
2. Place peppers and sweet potatoes in a freezer bag with vinegar and oil. Sprinkle with pepper and salt. Shake well.
3. Let it on a pan and roast for 30 minutes or till tender.
4. When the veggies are in the oven, place an iron skillet on medium heat.
5. Season your fish with pepper, salt and cumin.
6. Add olive oil in the skillet when it is hot. Fry the fillets till they get browned. Fry both sides till they can easily be lifted from the pan and the fish is cooked through.
7. Once the veggies are cooked. Remove from oven and place them in two plates.
8. Add spinach in the skillet. Stir till it gets wilted.
9. Place the fish on top of the veggies and serve hot.

COD and Cleric fries

Ingredients

Celeriac root – 1 (cut in ¼" strips)

Olive oil – 2 tbsp

Sea salt – to taste

Ground black pepper – to taste

Cod fillets – 1 lb

Lemon – 1

Arugula – 1 (small)

Olives – ½ cup (pitted)

Capers – 2 tbsp

Garlic – 2 cloves (chopped)

Instructions

1. Put your oven non preheat at 450°F
2. In an ovenproof dish, place the celeriac strips and drizzle with olive oil.
3. Top them with ground pepper and sea salt. Place them in the oven to bake for 10 minutes.
4. As the celeriac fries are baking, put cod fillets in another ovenproof dish. Top with lemon juice, ground pepper and sea salt.
5. Once the celeriac fried are done, lower the oven temperature to 400°Fand put the fish in the oven.
6. Bake the fish and fries together for 10 minutes.
7. In a food processor, add garlic, capers, olives and arugula. Blend well till it reaches the consistency of similar to a tapenade.
8. Pour this mixture on top of cod once it is baked.
9. Serve with celeriac fries on the side.

Pecans and Rosemary Salmon

Ingredients

Coconut oil – 2 tbsp

Salmon fillet – ¾ lb (skin on)

Pecans – 2 tbsp (chopped)

Rosemary – 1 tbsp (chopped)

Sea salt – ¼ tsp

Instructions

1. Put your oven on preheat at 350° F.
2. Top the fish with sea salt, rosemary and pecans.
3. Grease a baking dish with coconut oil and place the fish on it.
4. Put the baking dish in the oven for 15-20 minutes.

Veggies and Fish

Ingredients

Fish fillets – 1 lb (cut in 1" slices crosswise)

Coconut milk – 1 can

Red curry paste – 2 tbsp

Carrots – 2 (cut in strips)

Red cabbage – ½ (sliced)

Fresh cilantro – handful (chopped)

Instructions

1. In a large pan, mix together red curry paste and coconut milk. Cook over medium heat for 3-4 minutes and stir well.
2. Include red cabbage and carrots in the pan. Cover and let it cook for 5 minutes.
3. Afterwards add the fish in the mixture. Cook for another 5 minutes or until fish is cooked through.
4. Put the cooked fish on a clean plate and sprinkle with cilantro.
5. Serve.

Paleo Halibut

Ingredients

Coconut oil – 2 tbsp

Halibut – 1 lb

Dijon mustard – 2 tbsp

Almonds – 2 tbsp (chopped)

Instructions

1. Put your oven on preheat at 350 °F.
2. Grease a baking sheet with oil.
3. Place the fish skin side down on the baking sheet.
4. Pour Dijon mustard on the fish.
5. Top with almonds.
6. Place the fish in the oven for 15 minutes.
7. Serve warm.

Macadamia Fish

Ingredients

Fish fillets – 1 lb

Macadamia nuts – ¼ cup (halved)

Tomato – 1 (chopped)

Avocado – 1 (seeded and diced)

Fresh cilantro – 3 tbsp (chopped)

Fresh parsley – 3 tbsp (chopped)

Olive oil – 1 tbsp

Instructions

1. Put your grill on preheat.
2. Sprinkle the fish with ground pepper and sea salt.
3. Grill the fish for 4 minutes while turning it once.
4. In a bowl, add parsley, cilantro, avocado, tomatoes and macadamia. Mix them well and pour in olive oil for coating.
5. Serve the fish warm with salsa.

Azteca

Ingredients

Red snapper fillet – 1 lb

Lime juice – 1 lime

Lemon juice – ½ a lemon

Chili powder – 1 tsp

Tomato – 1 (chopped)

Green onions – 4 (sliced in ½" sections)

Anaheim pepper – 1 (chopped)

Red bell pepper – ½ (chopped)

Fresh cilantro – handful (chopped)

Instructions

1. In a baking dish, place the fillets.
2. Mix together chili powder, lemon juice and lime juice. Sprinkle this mixture on the fillets.
3. Leave for 10 minutes for marinating.
4. Put your oven on preheat at 350 °F.
5. Top the fillets with peppers, tomato and onions.
6. Cover the lid and let it bake for 30 minutes.
7. Leave it for about 4 minutes.
8. Sprinkle cilantro on top and serve.

Salmon and Lime

Ingredients

Salmon fillets – 1 lb (skinless)

Olive oil – 2 tbsp

Limes – 3 (halved)

Sea salt – ¼ tsp

Ground chipotle – ½ tsp

Instructions

1. Put your oven on preheat for 350 °F.
2. Place the salmon on a baking dish after cleaning and drying the fish.
3. Rub olive oil on each fillet and squeeze juice of half lime over each of them.
4. Top the fillets with chipotle and sea salt.
5. Put half lime over each fillet.
6. Bake for 15 minutes.
7. Serve warm.

Coconut Cream Salmon

Ingredients

Salmon fillet – 1 lb

Sea salt – ¼ tsp

Ground pepper – ¼ tsp

Coconut oil – 2 tsp

Shallot – 1 (diced)

Garlic – 3 cloves (minced)

Lemon zest – 1 lemon

Coconut milk – ½ cup

Fresh basil – 2 tbsp (chopped)

Instructions

1. Put your oven on preheat at 350 °F.
2. On a baking sheet, place the fillets and sprinkle them with pepper and salt on both sides.
3. On medium heat, place a sauté pan and add coconut oil in it once it is hot.
4. Add shallots and garlic and sauté them for 5 minutes or till they soften.
5. Include coconut milk, lemon juice and lemon zest in the mixture and let it boil.
6. Lower the heat and sprinkle with basil.
7. Pour this mixture on salmon fillets.
8. Bake for 20 minutes.
9. Serve.

Roasted Paleo Chicken

Ingredients

Sea salt – to taste

Ground black pepper – to taste

Fennel seeds – ¾ tsp (crushed)

Garlic powder – ¼ tsp

Dried oregano – ¼ tsp

Boneless chicken breasts – 4 (skinless)

Olive oil – 6 tbsp

Shallot – 1 (sliced thinly)

Fresh rosemary – 2 tsp (chopped)

Red bell peppers – 2 (sliced thinly)

Yellow bell pepper – 1 (sliced thinly)

Chicken broth – 1 cup

Balsamic vinegar – 1 tbsp

Instructions

1. Put your oven on preheat at 450 °F.
2. Mix together oregano, garlic powder, black ground pepper, fennel seeds and salt.
3. Rub chicken with spices and oil (2 tsp).
4. On medium high heat, place a large skillet and pour 2 tsp olive oil.
5. Include the chicken and let it cook for 3 minutes or till browned. Flip all the pieces and cook for another minute.
6. Transfer the chicken on a baking dish. Let it bake for 20 minutes or till cooked fully.
7. In the same skillet, pour in the rest of the oil at medium high heat.
8. Once hot, add rosemary and shallots. Sauté for 5 minutes or till translucent.
9. Include the chicken broth and peppers. Lower the heat and cook for 5 minutes.
10. Add in black pepper, salt and vinegar. Stir frequently and cook for 3 minutes.
11. Pour the sauce over the chicken
12. Serve hot.

Pineapples Peaches Chicken

Ingredients

Chicken – 3 lb (cut up)

Pineapple juice – 1 can

Fresh orange juice – 1 orange

Raisins – ½ cup

Almonds – ½ cup (sliced)

Cinnamon – ¼ tsp

Ground cloves – ¼ tsp

Ground black pepper – to taste

Pureed peaches (frozen or fresh) – 1 lb (sliced)

Instructions

1. Mix together cloves, cinnamon, almonds, raisins, orange juice, pineapple and chicken in skillet.
2. Cover the lid and let it simmer for 45 minutes. Stirring the chicken occasionally.
3. Include pureed peaches and mix well.
4. Uncover the lid and let it cook for 15 minutes or till the chicken is tender and the sauce is thick.
5. Transfer in a dish and sprinkle with black ground pepper.

Alla Griglia Paleo Chicken

Ingredients

Garlic – 2 tbsp (minced)

Vinegar – ½ cup

Cold water – 2 tbsp

Olive oil – ¼ cup

Raw honey – 1 tsp

Lemon – ½ (cut in ¼" slices)

Dried oregano – 1 tbsp

Dried rosemary – 1 tbsp

Red pepper flakes – ½ tsp

Sea salt – 1 tbsp

Boneless chicken – 1 (quartered)

Instructions

1. Except the chicken, mix together all the ingredients in a bowl.
2. In a large dish, place the chicken and pour the prepared sauce.
3. Leave it overnight to marinate.
4. During the next day, preheat your broiler at high heat.
5. Place chicken on a baking sheet.
6. On the roasting rack, put the baking sheet and let it broil for 5 minutes.
7. After wards, turn the temperature oven to 350 °F and bake the chicken for 20 minutes.
8. Serve hot with veggies.

Garlic Mushroom Chicken

Ingredients

Boneless chicken breasts – 1 lb (diced)

Olive oil – 2 tbsp

Sea salt – ½ tsp

Ground black pepper – ¼ tsp

Chili powder – ½ tsp

Garlic – 1 clove (minced)

Yellow onion – 1 (diced)

Mushrooms – 10 (sliced)

Red bell pepper – 2 (sliced)

Coconut milk – 1/3 cup

Instructions

1. In a bowl, mix together garlic, chili powder, black pepper, sea salt and olive oil (1tbsp). Cover and put in the refrigerator to marinate for an hour.
2. Before mealtime, place 2 skillets on medium heat.
3. Sauté the marinated chicken in one skillet till it is almost cooked.
4. In the other skillet, pour olive oil. Sauté onion for 5 minutes and put in the mushrooms. Cook till tender.
5. Add the chicken, coconut milk and red pepper, and stir well.
6. Let it cook for 10 minutes.
7. Serve hot.

Paleo Chicken Crusted

Ingredients

Eggs – 3 (beaten)

Water – 6 tbsp

Sea salt – ½ tsp

Ground black pepper – ¼ tsp

Almond flour – 1 cup

Boneless chicken breasts – 1 lb (skinless and cut each in 3 strips)

Instructions

1. Out your oven on preheat at 350 °F.
2. In a bowl, mix together water and eggs. Set aside.
3. In a plate, mix almond flour with black pepper and salt.
4. Dip the chicken strips in egg mixture and then in the almond flour on both sides.
5. To make the coating thicker, repeat the above-mentioned step.
6. In a baking sheet, place all the chicken strips and put it in the oven for 30-35 minutes.
7. Serve warm.

Paleo Yummilicious Steak

Ingredients

Beef flank steak – 1 lb

Olive oil – 1 tbsp

Chipotle powder – 1 tsp

Fresh pineapple – 4 slices

Red bell pepper – 1 (diced)

Red onion – ½ (diced)

Cilantro – ¼ cup (chopped)

Lime juice – 1 lime

Instructions

1. Heat the grill.
2. Mix together chipotle and oil in a dish. Brush this mixture on either sides of the steak.
3. Place the steak on grill and cook for 5 minutes on one side and 3 minutes on the other one.
4. Transfer the steak on a plate and side aside for 10 minutes. Ensure it is fully covered.
5. Next, place the pineapples on the grill and on each side grill for 3 minutes.
6. Once the pineapples are done, cut them into small chunks and place them in a bowl.
7. Include lime juice, cilantro, red onion and red bell pepper. Mix them well.
8. Cut the steak thin and serve with pineapple sauce.

Squash Spaghetti Lamb

Ingredients

Spaghetti squash – 1 (halved lengthwise)

Ground lamb – 1 lb

Ground liver – 1/8 lb

Yellow onion – ½ (diced)

Sea salt – ½ tsp

Garlic – ½ tsp

Oregano – ¼ tsp

Mushrooms – 8 (sliced)

Olive oil – 2 tbsp

Instructions

1. Put your oven on preheat at 375 °F.
2. Place the spaghetti squash (cut side down) in a baking dish. Pour water up to ¾" of the dish.
3. Bake the squash for 45 minutes.
4. Ina large pan, cook oregano, garlic, salt, onions, liver and lamb over medium high heat for 5 minutes. Stir frequently.
5. Include mushrooms in the mixture and let it cook for 12 minutes or till the lamb is cooked.
6. Once the squash is done, let it cool for a few minutes.
7. Turn the cut side up. With a fork, remove it from the rind. Ensure it is done cross wise.
8. Pour the sauce over the squash.
9. Serve hot.

Paleo Styled Meat Loaf

Ingredients

Dried sage – ¼ tsp

Seas slat – 1 tsp

Dry mustard – 1 tsp

Ground pepper – ½ tsp

Granulated garlic – 1 tsp

Chipotle chili powder – 1 tsp

Garlic – 4 cloves (chopped)

Yellow onion – 1 (chopped)

Red cabbage – 1 cup (chopped)

Coconut milk – 2 tbsp

Hot pepper sauce – ½ tsp

Almond meal – 1/3 cup

Egg- 1 (beaten)

Ground beef – 1-½ pounds

Instructions

1. Put oven on preheat at 350 °F.
2. Except ground beef, mix together all the ingredients in a bowl.
3. Once the ingredients are blended well, include the ground beef.
4. Put this mixture in a baking pan.
5. Bake for 85 minutes. Let it sit for 5 minutes.
6. Serve.

Classic Sloppy Joes - the Paleo Way

Ingredients

Ground beef – 1 lb

Olive oil – 2 tbsp

Onion – 1 (chopped)

Green pepper – 1 (chopped)

Garlic – 2 cloves (minced)

Tomato sauce – 1 can

Chili powder – 1 tbsp

Ground cumin – ½ tsp

Instructions

1. On medium heat, place a large skillet and add olive oil once it's hot.
2. Sauté garlic, green pepper and onion for 10 minutes or till tender.
3. Include ground beef.
4. Cook till meat turns brown for about 10 minutes while occasionally stirring.
5. Add ground cumin, chili powder and tomato sauce.
6. When the meat is cooked through, remove from heat.
7. Serve hot.

No Bun Burgers

Ingredients

Ground beef – 1 lb

Sea salt – ½ tsp

Ground black pepper – ¼ tsp

Coconut oil – 1 tsp

Instructions

1. Mix together salt and black pepper with the meat with the help of a fork.
2. Make four patties.
3. On medium heat, place a skillet and add coconut oil once it is hot.
4. Cook burgers till done.
5. Serve with grilled veggies.

Paleo Pork Dishes

Paleo Scrumptious Pizza

Ingredients

Almond flour – 1 cup

Almond butter – 3 tbsp

Eggs – 2

Sea salt – ½ tsp

Olive oil – 3 tsp

Yellow onion – ½ cup (diced)

Mushrooms – 4 (sliced)

Italian sausage – 1 (cut in ½" slices)

Garlic – 2 coves (minced)

Red pepper – 1 (diced)

Tomato sauce – ½ cup

Dried oregano – ½ tsp

Fennel seeds – ½ tsp

Grape tomatoes or cherry – ½ cup (halved)

Instructions

1. Put your oven on preheat at 350 °F.
2. In a bowl, mix together salt, eggs, almond butter and almond flour.
3. Sprinkle olive oil (2 tsp) on a baking sheet and spread the almond flour mixture on it. Make the crust ¼" thick.
4. Put the crust in the oven for 10 minutes.
5. In a skillet, add sliced sausage, mushrooms, onions and the rest of the olive oil. Cook on medium high heat or till sausage turn brown. Transfer in a bowl and set aside.
6. In the same skillet, sauté red pepper and garlic for a few minutes. Make sure the veggies don't get cooked completely as they will be baked with the pizza later.
7. Once the crust is done, spread tomato sauce all over it. Place the veggies and sausage slices on the pizza. Top with fennel seeds and oregano.
8. Bake for 30 minutes and once it is done tope with tomato slices.
9. Serve hot.

Paleo Pork Chops

Ingredients

Cayenne pepper – 2 tsp

Olive oil – 3 tbsp

Almond flour – 1½ cups

Pork chops – 4 (each 6 oz)

Instructions

1. In a shallow bowl, combine olive oil (2 tbsp) and cayenne pepper. Dip each pork chop in this mixture, making sure both sides are coated.
2. In a dish, place the almond flour and dip the pork chops in it till both sides on each pork chop are fully covered.
3. Put a skillet on medium heat; add olive oil (1 tbsp) once the skillet is hot.
4. Cook all the pork chops in the skillet till they are cooked through.
5. Serve.

Tomatoes and Sausage Combo

Ingredients

Tomatoes – 6

Pork Sausage – 1 lb

Mushrooms – 1 (sliced)

Yellow onion – 1 (chopped)

Fresh cilantro – handful

Instructions

1. Put your oven on preheat at 350 °F.
2. In a skillet, cook mushrooms, sausage and onions on medium high heat till they turn brown.
3. As the sausage mixture is cooking, remove the tomatoes' top. Remove the middle with the spoon and add in the skillet.
4. Once the mixture is done, drain the fat. With a spoon stuff the tomato cups with this mixture.
5. Place the tomatoes on a baking sheet and put in the oven.
6. Bake for 15 minutes.
7. Top with cilantro and serve.

Sausage and Veggies

Ingredients

Coconut oil – 2 tbsp

Leeks – 3 (chopped)

Seasoned ground pork sausage – 1 lb

Fire roasted crushed tomatoes – 1 can (28 oz)

Lemon juice – ½ lemon

Italian seasoning – 2 tbsp

Granulated garlic – ½ tsp

Red pepper flakes – ½ tsp

Cauliflower head – 1 (only florets)

Instructions

1. Place a pan on medium high heat and once it is hot, add coconut oil and leeks. Sauté for 5 minutes.
2. Include the sausage and let it cook till it is fully done.
3. Add red pepper flakes, lemon, garlic, Italian seasoning and tomatoes. Cook for 20 minutes on medium heat. Stir occasionally.
4. Put the cauliflower in microwave and set the time for 5 minutes. Next, blend it in a food processor till it reaches rice like consistency.
5. Top the sausage mixture with salt and spoon it over the cauliflower.
6. Serve warm.

Sausages with Artichokes

Ingredients

Pork Sausage – 1 lb

Olive oil – 2 tbsp

Onions – 2 (cut in thick segments)

Garlic – 1 clove (sliced finely)

Mushrooms – 5 (halved)

Jerusalem artichokes – ½ lb (scrubbed and cut in 1" pieces)

Lemon – ½ (cut in large chunks)

Fennel seeds – ½ tsp

Water – 1 cup

Flat leaf parsley – small bunch (chopped)

Steamed spring cabbage or kale – to serve

Instructions

1. In a deep cast iron skillet, cook the sausage with little oil. Remove from skillet and set aside.
2. In the same skillet add onions. Let them cook for 20 minutes or till they are tender and can be easily crushed with a wooden spoon.
3. Include the garlic, mushrooms and artichokes in the skillet. Let them cook till the artichokes color slightly.
4. Add the cooked sausage in the skillet. Include pepper, salt, funnel seeds and lemon.
5. Pour in enough water in the skillet to cover the mixture.
6. When the water comes to a boil, lower the heat and let it cook for 30 minutes or till veggies are tender.
7. If there is still too much water left, turn the heat to high and let it reduce.
8. Top with parsley and serve with steamed spring cabbage or kale.

Paleo Special Baked Ice Cream

Ingredients

Bananas – 2 (ripe)

Coconut ice cream – 2 scoops

Ground cinnamon – ½ tsp

Instructions

1. Put the oven on preheat at 350 °F.
2. In a dish, place the bananas and bake them for 30 minutes or till soft.
3. Squeeze out the bananas in two plates and top them with 1 scoop of ice cream each.
4. Sprinkle with cinnamon and serve.

Roll Up Fruits

Ingredients

Apples – 2

Strawberries – 2 (remove the greens)

Cinnamon – 1 tsp

Water – ¼ cup

Instructions

1. Dice and core apples.
2. Blend together, cinnamon, water, strawberries and apples in a blender. Process for 30 seconds or till smooth.
3. On a Teflex sheet, pour and spread the mixture. Place the sheet in plastic dehydrator. Leave for 6-8 hours.
4. Remove Teflex and switch the sides of the fruits.
5. Continue to dehydrate for another 6 hours.

Paleo Scrumptious Cookies

Ingredients

Almond flour – 3 cups

Coconut oil – ½ cup

Raw honey – ½ cup

Eggs – 2

Baking soda – 1 tsp

Sea salt – 1 tsp

Vanilla extract – 1 tsp

Semi-sweet chocolate chips – 1 ½ cups

Instructions

1. Put oven on preheat at 375 °F and place parchment paper on baking sheet.
2. In a bowl, mix together salt, baking soda and almond flour. Set aside.
3. In another bowl, add vanilla extract, honey and eggs. Beat with a mixer.
4. Pour this mixture slowly in the almond flour mixture. Blend them well. Add the chocolate chips.
5. Spoon gold ball sized dough on the baking sheet. Make sure there is a 2" gap between all the cookies.
6. Place in the oven and bake for 10 minutes.

Apple Pie

Ingredients

<u>For Crust:</u>

Sunflower seeds – 1 ½ cup

Raisins – ¾ cup

Carob powder – 1 tbsp

<u>For Filling:</u>

Apples – 6 (peeled and cored)

Raw honey – ¾ cup

Cinnamon – 1 tbsp

Lemon juice – ½ lemon

Shredded coconut – ¼ cup

Instructions

1. In a food processor, add carob powder, raisins and sunflower seeds. Blend till finely ground.
2. In a pie pan, spread the crust.
3. Place the apples in the food processor. Pulse them until they are small chunks.
4. Mix together honey, lemon juice, cinnamon and apples in a bowl.
5. Spread this mixture over the crust. Save the juice that remains in the bowl.
6. Level the mixture on the crust and top with coconut flakes.
7. Refrigerate for 1 hour or till the pie is set.
8. Serve.

Sweet Paleo Bars

Ingredients

Olive oil – 3 tbsp

Carob powder – ¼ cup

Groundnuts – ½ cup

Shredded coconut – ¾ cup

Raw honey – 1 tbsp

Instructions

1. Cook together, olive oil and honey in a pan at low heat for 3-4 minutes. Take off from heat.
2. Add coconut, groundnuts and carob powder in it. Mix well.
3. Cover a baking sheet with parchment paper. Pour the mixture over the paper.
4. Once it is cool enough, form any shape you want.
5. Refrigerate until hardened.
6. Cut into slices and serve.

Final Words

Healthy eating habits ensure a better life. Paleo diet is a perfect way to ensure you and your loved one stay fit and strong. With these 50 scrumptious Paleo recipes, you won't feel any craving for junk food, as each one of these recipes is sure to satiate your hunger. Have fun making these recipes and don't forget to experiment with different ingredients. Use your creativity and you will end up with another delicious meal.

Made in the USA
Las Vegas, NV
23 October 2021